I0122682

COPYRIGHT

Copyright © 2025 by Lisa Ellis
All Rights Reserved.
No part of this publication may be reproduced,
distributed, or transmitted in any form or by any means, including
photocopying, recording, or other electronic or mechanical methods,
or by any information storage and retrieval system without the prior
written permission of the publisher, except in the case of very brief
quotations embodied in critical reviews and certain other
noncommercial uses permitted by copyright law.

DISCLAIMER

This book reflects my personal experiences, insights, and journey with cancer. It is intended for informational, inspirational, and educational purposes only. Anything contained within its pages should not be considered medical advice. I am not a licensed medical or mental health professional.
Always consult a qualified healthcare provider for
medical advice. Everyone is unique. What worked for me may not work for you. The 5 Secrets shared within this book are based on my personal experience battling
cancer and the shakeup on my life that ensued.

INTRODUCTION

You've Been Given Another Chance

I never thought cancer would be a part of *my* story. I was younger than the average person who was diagnosed with endometrial adenocarcinoma. Simply put, my female parts – designed to give life, were now trying to take mine.

I had always been healthy — the kind of healthy that annoys friends. No major injuries. Only two minor surgeries my whole life. Nearly every medical test I'd ever taken came back perfectly normal. Until, one day, the test didn't.

I had just moved into what my husband and I called our "dream home build." You know that season when life feels like dreams are finally materializing? Boxes were barely unpacked, the house still smelled new-house fresh, and we were figuring out where to place our stuff in our new space. Then came the news that would flip everything upside down: cancer.

To make cancer even more interesting, we had just moved to a brand-new area. No local doctors. No medical history on file. And, as if that wasn't enough, no health insurance. I sometimes joke that if life were a board game, this was the point where someone swiped half my game pieces off the board and said, "Let me know how that works out for you!"

But cancer doesn't really care if you're too young. It doesn't care if you've been healthy your whole life. It doesn't care that you're currently living your best HGTV moment in your dream home. It just shows up. Uninvited. And, very suddenly your world gets divided into "before" and "after."

The "before" me thought health was something I could take for granted. The "after" me knows health is something I *fight* for. The "before" me thought my life was on track, under control. The "after" me knows control is mostly an illusion — but courage, laughter, and love are not.

This book is for the "after" you. The version of you who has walked through something terrifying, exhausting, and life-altering… and now looks around and wonders, *What do I do with this life I still have?*

I won't pretend to have all the answers. What I do have are 5 secrets — simple but powerful ways to heal, to laugh again, and to give yourself permission to truly live after cancer. These secrets aren't about perfection. They're about progress, perspective, and maybe even a few good punchlines along the way.

Because here's your reality: you didn't survive cancer just to live a smaller life. You survived for something bigger, brighter, and bolder. And you don't need anyone's permission to step into that… except maybe your own.

So consider this book your permission slip. Your invitation to rebuild, to reimagine, and to rejoice in the life you still have. Healing may not look like a straight line, but I promise you this: it can be filled with hope, humor, and heart.

Let's get started.

ABOUT THE AUTHOR

ABOUT THE AUTHOR:

Lisa Ellis is a cancer survivor, thriver, and advocate for women learning to live fully again after diagnosis. At a younger-than-average age and with almost no risk
factors, she was stunned by her cancer diagnosis. The diagnosis was made even more difficult as she had just moved to a new city, had no family or friends nearby, and no health insurance. Today, 1.5 years cancer-free, she shares her story to help other women find courage, laughter, and freedom on the other side of survival.

Blending honesty, hope, and humor, she offers practical tools for overcoming fear, healing mind–body–spirit, and daring to dream big *again*. She lives in South Florida with her husband and finds joy in exploring the outdoors, writing, and reminding women everywhere that life after cancer is worth living.

For Karl — my rock, my partner, my best friend through the storm.
For my family and friends, who showed up, held space, offered prayers, made me laugh, let me cry, and reminded me I was *NEVER* alone.
And for my fellow survivors — you are my inspiration, my mirror, and my motivation to rise again.

WHY READ THIS BOOK?

Fear IS Real

My Personal Story

I wasn't the typical candidate for my type of cancer. From six possible risk factors, I checked *EXACTLY* one. My husband and I had just moved into our dream home in a new city—no doctors nearby, no friends or family close, and no support system. I'd been healthy most of my life. Hardly ever needed medical care, other than annual check ups. And to make matters worse, I had no health insurance.

In a matter of days, my world shifted from "normal" to navigating doctor visits, medical test jargon, and the terrifying unknown. Maybe you know that feeling—when life turns upside down and nothing feels safe anymore.

Identifying the Problem

In reality, surviving cancer is a beginning. Many women find themselves stuck in fear—fear of recurrence, fear of death, fear of never living fully again. Instead of reclaiming life, they find themselves trapped in a cycle of anxiety and exhaustion.

The Reality: A Bigger Problem Than We Think

Did you know that studies show **more than 59% of cancer survivors experience ongoing fear of recurrence**? And nearly **1 in**

3 report feeling more anxious after treatment ends than they did during it. Cancer may end, but the emotional toll can linger long after your last appointment.

My Mission and Passion

I know this journey because I've lived it. That's why I wrote this book—for women like you who want more than just "survival." I believe with every ounce of my being that there is life *after* cancer—life filled with joy, connection, and dreams worth chasing. For the record, I am a little over a year and a half cancer free at the time of this writing.

And as a survivor, author, and advocate, my mission is to guide you out of fear and into freedom, offering tools I've personally tested in my own healing journey.

The Promise of This Book

In these pages, I'll share with you **five powerful secrets to living fully beyond cancer.** You'll discover not just how to cope, but how to thrive.

This book will help you:

1. Move beyond the fear of looming death.
2. Reclaim your identity outside of cancer.
3. Step into a life filled with laughter, hope, and heart.

The Benefits You'll Gain

By the time you finish this book, you'll know how to:

Craft joy – Build daily practices that help you embrace life with gratitude and lightness.

Build a support team – Surround yourself with people who lift you up and walk this path beside you.

Dream big – Give yourself permission to pursue bold new dreams and passions, no matter where you are in your journey.

Why You Can't Afford to Wait

Here's the hard truth: every day you let fear and uncertainty rule your life is another day of loss. The longer you wait to reclaim your joy, the harder it becomes to break free from anxiety and "just surviving." You deserve to live fully—not someday, but now. Cancer free.

Read On…

This is your invitation—your permission—to start living again. Five secrets have the power to transform how you see yourself, your future, and your life beyond cancer. In the chapters ahead, you'll discover not only guidance and practical steps but also a renewed sense of hope, humor, and heart.

Are you ready?

Let's begin.

SECRET 1 - DO YOUR PART

Healing Your Mind, Body, and Spirit

When your cancer treatment ends, people feel that the hard part is finally over. Reality check: your part of the healing process begins when your cancer treatment ends.

The Myth of "All Better"

The day my treatment ended, people congratulated me like I had just finished a marathon. "You must feel so relieved! You must be so happy it's all behind you now!"

At first, I wasn't sure how to respond. I wanted to say: *"Yes, except my body feels like it's revolting, my brain is buzzing with every 'what if' death scenario possible, and my emotions fluctuate among weepy, grateful, and angry."*

Here's what most people don't understand: healing doesn't end when treatment does. In some ways, ending treatment is the beginning. Doctors can remove tumors and prescribe medicine, but they can't fix exhaustion, fear of recurrence, or the way your body feels like it's no longer the one you used to know. That part is up to you — and that's where Secret 1 comes into play.

Healing is a partnership. The doctors do their part. Now it's time for you to do yours.

Healing Your Mind

Cancer messes with your head. One minute you're fine, the next minute you're spiraling because you sneezed twice in a row and wonder if it's a symptom. (Spoiler: it's probably just allergies.)

For me, my mind, body, and spirit became totally divergent. My mind said *I can't handle this – so, I'm just going to ignore it.* My body said *Freak-out-mode activated!* And my spirit actively wondered if it was time to join my ancestors.

I discovered healing your mind is about learning to catch those spirals, preventing them from robbing you of happiness.

A few tricks that rescued me from the spiral:

Name it out loud. Sometimes saying, *"That's just scanxiety talking,"* helps quiet the voice. Tell yourself, *"Today, I'm ok."* Let the feeling of being OK enter your body. Hold onto that feeling.

Talk to someone. A counselor, support group, or even a trusted friend can help you reframe what's swirling in your head. True story: I joined a support group about a month after my tumor was removed. (Yeah, I know. It took me a month to get there. Do it in your own time. You'll know when you're ready.) I was so nervous about the support group that I completely *missed* a tornado warning which cancelled the group meeting. I drove an hour through pouring rain, lightning – you get the picture. When I discovered the meeting was cancelled, I started tearing up. The lady who hosted the group, a breast cancer survivor, realized I needed help. So, she met with me – by myself for one hour! That one hour helped calm my mind and put me on a new path to healing. I began to realize that death was not eminent.

Write it down. When you mind becomes divergent, write it down. I remember realizing that my mind was focused on other things and I wasn't remembering things I was doing that were habit. You know, little things – paying insurance, the gas bill, etc. I discovered that writing things down helped focus my mind on everyday tasks and quieted the part that was obsessed with my diagnosis.

Find your sense of humor. I kept a mental file of funny things people said to me — like the friend who tried to comfort me by saying, *"At least you won't have periods anymore."* Or my sister, who when I boldly told her "I'm going to take up skydiving" reminded me of the nagging fact that I'm afraid of heights. As an alternative, she
suggested *"I should have Karl push me off the bed. See how I deal with falling from that high BEFORE I take up skydiving."* Not helpful, but definitely funny.

Healing Your Body

Let's be honest: your body after cancer feels like something from a freak-show. It's still you, but… not quite.

I had always been healthy — never anything more than two surgeries in my life. But after treatment, I felt like my body was secretly plotting additional ways to kill me. Some days I had energy, other days it felt like I was
wading through mud.

Healing your body is about patience and listening:

Rest without guilt. Fatigue is not laziness. It's your body rebuilding. Remind yourself to take time to heal. If it's not an emergency, it can wait.

Move gently. Yoga, walking, stretching — think of it as reminding your body how to feel alive again. Enjoying walks in nature reconnect you with the beauty surrounding you.

Feed your body with kindness. This doesn't mean kale smoothies every day (though God bless you if that's your thing). It means foods that nourish and don't leave you feeling worse. Discover food that nourishes your body.

And yes, naps! I count them as exercise. At least in my book.

Healing Your Spirit

This part looks different for everyone, but it's often the most overlooked. When cancer steals your sense of safety, you need something bigger to root yourself in.

For some, that's faith. For others, it's meditation, gratitude, or simply spending time in nature. My spirit started healing in the quiet moments — sipping coffee in the morning sun with my husband, watching a sunset, or noticing the ordinary daily things I used to rush past.

The point is, your spirit needs just as much care as your body and mind. Find what lifts you. Do it often. If someone offers to pray for you, say *YES*!

Your Healing Game Plan

Healing doesn't happen by accident. It happens by intention. That's why I encourage you to create a simple "Healing Game Plan."

Here's what mine looked like:

Mind: Focus on 1 thing a day to facilitate healing.

Body: Move my body. Walk. Go to the grocery story. Get out of the house. Schedule 20 minutes every day.

Spirit: Start mornings with one thing I'm grateful for. Here's mine. Say it aloud, *"I'm grateful for my life and my family."*

It wasn't perfect. Some days I skipped all of it. But over time, those small things rebuilt me. Make choices which heal you.

The Humor in Healing

Healing will never be tidy. Some days you'll feel strong, other days you'll cry in the grocery store because you're overwhelmed by the music playing. (True story.) The key is to give yourself grace — and maybe a laugh.

Once, I fell asleep mid-conversation during a phone call to schedule follow up appointments. Making matters worse, it was moments after declaring I "wasn't even tired." (Luckily my husband rescued the call.) Instead of being embarrassed, I let it become part of my story.

Because if cancer taught me anything, it's that life is too short not to laugh at yourself.

Takeaway: Do Your Part

Healing isn't passive.

It's not just waiting for your body to catch up.

It's saying:

I will care for my mind.

I will honor my body.

I will nurture my spirit.

And I'll do it one small step, one small laugh, one small act of grace at a time.

Because healing isn't about becoming the old you again. It's about becoming the *new you* — stronger, softer, wiser, and maybe even a little saucier.

SECRET 2 - LIMITLESS LIFE

Refuse to Downgrade Your Future

After cancer, everyone suddenly becomes the spokesperson for your "new normal." (Did I mention I despise that term?) It sounds like a consolation prize for surviving — a gentle pat on the head followed by, *"Sorry, kid. You could have been this, but now you're going to have to settle for that."* When did surviving become synonymous with "accept less?"

Believe me when I tell you this simple fact:

Your life isn't a downgrade unless you choose to downgrade it.

Refusing the Downgrade

After cancer, shrinking feels safe. Playing small feels responsible. Dreaming big feels crazy — like you're tempting fate. And honestly? I experienced days when disappearing from my own life felt easier than rebuilding it.

I nearly sold everything and sailed off into the sunset just to escape the pressure of figuring out what the next version of me looks like. Then reality set in: I'm a white-knuckled sailor who gets anxious when the wind shifts the wrong way. Sailing off into the sunset wasn't an option.

I came to realize that cancer took a lot from me, but I didn't have to willingly hand over the rest of me. And, dear reader, **neither do you**.

Even when treatment is over, cancer leaves mental landmines everywhere — doubt, fear, fragility,

hyper-awareness of every *different* sensation. Suddenly your dreams feel too loud, too risky, too *much*. Like your pushing your luck. But the future you've earned isn't built by tiptoeing around what you've experienced.

Limiting Belief Busting
Let's get honest: **your body is forever changed.**

That's not negative — it's reality.
But *changed* does not equal *broken.*
And *different* does not equal *diminished.*

You're allowed to grieve what you lost. I did. I missed the ease, the energy, the version of myself who didn't   overthink every ache. But grief is a place to visit — not a place to take up permanent residence.

At my first post-op appointment, barely a week after surgery, my doctor looked at me and said, "You should get back to walking five miles, three times a week. There's no reason you can't."

I stared at him. I had just mastered the art of getting out of bed without wincing. Five miles??? I wanted to ask if he'd like to try that with stitches tugging at his insides.

But underneath all of that was a quiet whisper: *What if he's right? What if I can?*

The next morning, I laced up my shoes and walked. Not five miles — just half a mile to the recreation center. It was slow. It was uncomfortable. But it was a start. And by the end of the week, I was hitting small targets. Not gracefully. Not without effort. But consistently.

And then — one day — I walked five miles again.

What changed?

My perspective.

I stopped saying *"I can't"* and started asking, *"Why can't I?"*

When you feel stuck, scared, or triggered by the memory of your diagnosis, remind yourself:

You don't go "back." You go forward.

Designing Your Future

Now let's talk about what comes next. *Survival?* You've done that. *Settling for less?* NO! *Shrinking your life because you're afraid to want more?* You don't have to – shrinking is a choice.

Ask yourself the question most people avoid:

"What do I want my cured life to look like?"

Not "manageable."

Not "safe."

Not "acceptable for someone who's been through a lot."

What do *you* want?

Grab a pen. It's time to design your future — not get pushed into it.

Step 1 — Curate Your Future

Write down **five things** you want to accomplish after cancer. Uncensored answers. Pick goals that challenge you.

Here were mine:
Eat healthier
Lose weight
Publish a book
Develop an online course
Buy another rental property

These weren't just goals. They were evidence that my dreams didn't die just because cancer tried to rewrite my story.

Step 2 — Add Small Actionable Items

Big dreams require tiny, achievable steps. List **three small actions** beneath each of your five goals. At least one should be so easy you can do it today. Who doesn't like quick wins, right?

Here's my example:
Goal: Eat healthier

Action steps:
Limit refined sugars
Learn about nutrition after cancer
Find healthy recipes that won't bore me; try one new recipe per week.

Small steps create momentum. And momentum builds belief that you *CAN* reach your goals.

Step 3 — Re-evaluate

After a week or two, pause and check in:

What worked?

What didn't?

Where did fear slip back in?

Where did you surprise yourself?

You're not just healing your body — you're reacquainting yourself with who you are now.

Step 4 — Refine Your Plan
Adjust. Update. Rewrite. Remove. Add.

Do whatever you need to create a life that feels like it belongs to *you* — not your diagnosis.

A limitless life isn't built in one dramatic moment.

It's built through a series of brave, imperfect steps from a person who refuses to accept a downgraded version of their future.

Takeaway: Do Your Part
No one can rebuild your life for you.

People can support you, cheer for you, and walk alongside you.

But the rebuilding?

The mindset shift?

The courageous choosing?

That part is yours.

Say this with me:
I refuse to downgrade my future.

I will create a life that excites me.

I will actively pursue the dreams cancer tried to steal.

Cancer changed your story — but it does not get to write the ending.

You do!

SECRET 3 - CRAFT JOY

Laugh Loud, Live Loud

Cancer doesn't exactly come with a punchline. There's nothing funny about fear, sleepless nights, or the endless appointments. But once you've experienced trial by fire, you embrace a strange kind of wisdom — one that
whispers, *"Laughter really does heal."*

Crafting joy isn't about pretending cancer never
happened. It's about refusing to let fear or sadness rule your world. When you genuinely laugh loud, you live loud.

After everything you've been through, <u>let's agree you've earned both.</u>

Why Humor Is Body and Soul Medicine

You don't have to be a medical professional to know that real laughter changes you. Think about your last genuine laugh. It ripples through your chest, your shoulders drop (or maybe shake uncontrollably like mine), and for one triumphant moment, your body owns peace. And,
science agrees. Laughter works inside you to your benefit.

Let's talk about why. Laughter boosts oxygen flow,
massages your lungs and heart, and releases endorphins — natural happy, feel-good chemicals. Endorphins
counteract stress hormones like cortisol and adrenaline, resulting in a more relaxed and centered you (Mayo Clinic, 2023)!

Researchers discovered laughter stimulates circulation and aids muscle relaxation. The result – reduced stress. I like to call it nature's built-in reset button. That may even explain the recent uptick in yoga laughter sessions. . . or not.

Of course, laughter is not a cure. It's comfort. A reminder to breathe, laugh, and reset. Light still finds its way into life.

And that's what laughter does best – reminds you that it's ok to find humor in life – even in the messy parts.

Permission to Enjoy Life Again (Minus Guilt)

Surviving cancer doesn't mean you automatically wake up joyful. If anything, you wake up cautious – looking for signs that you're actually cured. Understandable, you've spent months — maybe years — preparing for the next test, the next scan, the next "what if" scenario dancing in your mind.

When happiness shows up, it can feel . . . strange.

Can I laugh again? Attend a concert? Plan a trip when my doctor is a 10 hour airplane ride away?

YES! YOU CAN!

Reclaiming joy isn't betraying what you've survived — it's honoring it. It's the proof that you are still here – to live.

Psychologists call this "post-traumatic growth." Let's put that in beautifully simple terms: out of hardship, new appreciation develops. Cancer survivors shift into appreciation for life. Relationships deepen, gratitude grows, priorities sharpen – eliminating things which no longer spark joy.

So here's your permission slip, written in invisible ink across your scars: **YOU ARE ALLOWED TO ENJOY LIFE AGAIN.**

Guilt-free. Unapologetically. Without fearing the next
result.

Create Your Joy List

Joy doesn't always arrive in grand gestures. Most days, it's a flicker
— a moment you make on purpose. Think of your Joy List as
physical therapy for your spirit: small, repeatable motions that help
you reclaim your range of motion in life.

Here's how to start:

Set a tiny goal. Ten minutes a day of something that feels good. Not
forced good — *real* good.

Brain-dump the little things. Write down every simple joy you can
think of. Don't edit. Don't justify. Just list.

A few examples:
A kitchen dance party with your favorite song
Sending a funny cat meme to your bestie
Warm towels straight from the dryer
A sunset walk, if you're like me – preferably near water
Your favorite laugh-out-loud podcast while waiting in traffic
A slice of apple that tastes crisp like fall

Make it visible. Stick it on your mirror, fridge, or phone wallpaper.

Put it on the calendar. Yes, joy deserves a time slot too. Craft time
to make joy and recognize it.

Notice how you feel. Afterward, take a breath and ask yourself, *Do I
feel better?*

Want to Recover Like a Pro? Create a "Laugh Kit."

Save three videos, one podcast episode, and one photo that make you
genuinely laugh. Look at them on your next hard day. Flip the

switch. When your mind says, "Nothing will help," you'll have proof it's wrong.

Joy doesn't erase pain — it simply reminds you that you can choose to *feel* something else.

Live Loud (Without Being 'That Loud')

"Living loud" isn't about being obnoxious or dramatic. It's about refusing to crawl into a corner.

When you live loud, you speak your needs, you ask tough questions, and you realize life is colorful again. You stop whimpering and feeling bad for yourself. You stop apologizing for surviving.

Living loud can include things like:

Wearing the brightest scarf you own to your doctor's appointment, just because you like it.

Laughing too loudly at a coffee shop, unbothered by whether or not it's appropriate.

Taking a weekend trip just because the world is still beautiful and *YOU CAN*!

Saying "no" to what exhausts you and "yes" to what empowers you.

It's not about faking joy. It's about embodying it.

Because after cancer, quiet survival is no longer an option — you deserve full-volume living.

Try This: The "Live Loud" Exercise

Pick your passion. What's one place you've been shrinking — a dream, a hobby, a decision you keep deferring?

Amp up the volume one notch. Choose a passion — just one.

A few examples:
Share your writing passion with a friend. (I'm doing that right now!)
Say yes to the invitation to that kickboxing class.
Take the picture, even if your hair hasn't quite grown back yet.

Add a laugh. Pair your courage with something silly — a playlist, a meme, or crafting a breakfast opera (you can ask my husband about this one).

Reflect. How did it feel to amp up the volume of your authentic self (even if it was just for a moment)?

This isn't about ignoring what happened to you — it's about making sure you continue live your best life
forward.

The Takeaway
Joy doesn't mean denial.

It means you're choosing to live fully, even when you get tested by life.

Laughter is your body's rebellion against fear. It's proof you're still here — healing with hope, humor, and heart.

Craft your joy on purpose. Laugh loud. Live loud.

Because life after cancer isn't about being quietly grateful.

It's about being unapologetically alive.

Live Loud Reflection Worksheet

An exercise to help you step back into your full, fearless, and joyful self.

Let's boldly take one small, brave step to reflect.

Step 1: Identify Your Fears

Where have you been holding back or playing small?

_____

_____

_____

_____

Step 2: Turn Up the Volume

Identify one small way you can turn up the volume and sprinkle fun on your life this week?

It could be as simple as wearing bright colors, speaking up, or saying yes to something.

_____

_____

_____

Step 3: Add a Laugh

How can you bring humor or lightness into your world this moment?

Think of a funny song, silly video, or fun friend.

_____

_____

_____

Step 4: Reflection

How did if feel to show up as your fullest, loudest, most alive-self-moment?

_____

_____

_____

Step 5: Boldly Declare Out Loud

Today I choose to live loud.

To be fully, bravely, and beautifully me.

I will laugh, love, and live.

SECRET 4 - HEALING HAPPENS TOGETHER

Because Healing Doesn't End When Treatment Does

When treatment ends, congratulations begin. You're left with an odd feeling that mixes gratitude with dread. Gratitude comes from the realization that the hardest parts of treatment are over. While dread creeps in
because you realize you have a 5-year window of follow up appointments which include rescreening for cancer at specific intervals. You should walk out into the sunshine ready to begin life anew, right? Yet, this cloud hovers over your head. Life after cancer isn't a simple switch flip
setting life "back to normal."

Normal has changed.

Your body's healing. You're getting back to routine but the cloud refuses to dissipate. The reality? Healing doesn't end when treatment does—it just takes a
different form. And you're not meant to heal alone.

So, how can you forget about that nagging cloud and keep living? That's what we're going to talk about in this section.

The Myth of "I'm Fine"

When the treatments stop, the silence can be deafening.

Support networks of family and friends go back to their routines. You tell them you're "fine" because you desperately *want* to be fine. You want to believe it's over. The rescreening part is "just routine" and "no big deal."

But deep down, you know healing is more than physical. It's emotional, spiritual, and relational. Even the strongest survivors need people who keep showing up—this time, not with medical charts and tests, but with your favorite coffee, jokes, love, patience, and sometimes - dinner!

You need a team. A team not helping you *fight* —but one reminding you to *live.*

The Bounce-Back Bunch
Introducing *The Bounce-Back Bunch.*

Think of *The Bounce-Back Bunch* like your own personal circle of superheroes. Friends and family who remind you that you are more than your cancer. They show up with hope, humor, and heart — lightening your load on the heavy days while adding laughter and joy when words fall short.

They help you find your strength again - sometimes with a push, other times walking beside you while holding your hand. The Bounce-Back Bunch celebrates small victories, reminds you to heal, and reflects back the courage you might forget you possess.

With them, healing becomes tangible – a celebration of life, love, and the incredible power of coming back stronger than before.

For me, my Bounce-Back Bunch showed up in ways I never expected. My husband refused to let me sink into self-pity, even when I felt like giving in to it. My sister filled my days with laughter, the kind that bubbles up and reminds you of the times when life was simple. My brother listened — really listened — without judgment, letting me process messy emotions that don't fit neatly into ordinary conversation. My friends and neighbors went shopping, brought food, and gently nudged me back into living — even encouraging me to take that first trip I was too afraid to plan.

Perhaps the most unexpected Bounce-Back Bunch
member was my surgeon. His dry humor somehow made the hard parts bearable. He'd say things like, "Well, that's better than dead," not to dismiss my struggle but to
remind me, in the most human way, that life was still mine to live. He took my calls, calmed my fears, and somehow showed compassion while doing all of these things.

Combine all of these small moments — the laughter, the listening, the care, the unexpected humor — and you discover you have something powerful. Their support
reminded me that yes, life had changed, but it wasn't over. I could still accomplish anything I set my mind to and there was still opportunity in life.

When you let people in, you might be surprised who shows up for you. I learned that trusting others with my life gave me a quiet kind of strength — the kind that whispers, *"If all these people believe I can survive, maybe I can believe it too."*

Letting people in didn't make me weaker. It actually did the opposite - it made me unstoppable. Life reminded me that healing isn't meant to be done alone — you heal through connection, courage, and trust. My Bounce-Back Bunch reminded me that every setback offers the opportunity for a comeback. Every act of kindness is a spark that fuels the will to keep it together and keep going. Together, we proved that healing isn't just about getting back to who you were — it's about becoming someone even stronger, braver, and more alive than
before.

Because when you let others lift you, you discover just how high you were meant to rise.

Reflection Time

Who are your Bounce-Back Bunch people?
Choose at least 3 people that make you feel most alive.

How can you let them help you heal?

SECRET 5 - LIVE BOLDLY

Give Yourself Permission to Dream Again

Surviving cancer isn't the finish line. Think of survival as the starting gun for your second chance at life. Now, ask yourself: *Did you come this far to retreat and live small or do you want more?*

When I was first diagnosed with cancer, I remember walking into my first oncology appointment. The room was filled with patients. I examined their faces and thought: *Do they look like they have cancer? Do I look like I have cancer? Am I going to die?*

I was shaken to my core. My picture-perfect life evaporated in that instance.

Now that I am cancer free, I still see the faces of the women. I wonder how many of them survived. My mind then slips into fear, maybe even panic. *How many of them thought they were cancer free and got it AGAIN?*

You will also feel that fear. Fear of recurrence. Fear of death. Guess what? That's called being human. You're normal. I am here to tell you that you can still step into life boldly. Let me show you how.

Reclaiming Postponed Dreams

What did you want to do before you were diagnosed?

Did you want to get a college degree? Take a trip?
Reconnect with old friends?

Think hard about this one. Take a moment. Jot it down.

My postponed dream was getting back into shape. I have always
been on the heavier side and wanted to loose some weight. My
husband and I had just started exercising regularly when I was
diagnosed. And, I am a stress eater – I think you know where I am
going with this one.
Needless to say I put on weight because I was stressed. Now that I
was cancer free and my physical scars were healing, I knew it was
time to do something.

In fact, I asked my surgeon how I could avoid getting
cancer again. He said words I'll never forget. "Lose weight. The type
of cancer you had loves fat. And, stay away from anything with
soy." Ok. Sounds simple enough. But not exactly motivating. So,
how do you get motivated?

Here's the secret – whatever you want to do, break it down into
smaller parts. I wanted to lose weight, but I was also restricted
during my recovery due to surgery. I knew I couldn't just go out and
walk 5 miles. I had to build up to it. So, I decided to walk to the
mailbox – for the record the mailbox is a couple blocks away, not at
the end of my driveway. After about a week, I was able to easily do
that.

I celebrated my little victory. Then, I pushed myself to go further.
The next week my goal was to walk 1 mile. After about another
week, I could easily do that.

I celebrated my latest victory. Then, I pushed myself to go further.
The next week my goal was to walk 3.5 miles. Three days later, I
could do that too!

Another victory to celebrate! More momentum. And then I added new exercises.

My point, you *CAN* still accomplish what you desire. Just break it down into smaller parts and move on it.

Risks, Adventures, & New Passions

Now, time for more risky stuff. I thought about skydiving . . . Well, my sister successfully talked me out of that one. However, one thing was still on my list that was risky – INTERNATIONAL TRAVEL.

I really wanted to travel abroad but there was a *HUGE* piece of me that was scared-to-death about being a 10 hour flight away from my doctors. Not to mention the fact that I was now immunocompromised and would be around a bunch of microbes, trapped in a confined space with recirculated air – TOTAL FREAK OUT.

Honestly, it didn't have to be a total freak out. I asked myself, *What would make me feel better about this?* The answer – buy international health insurance! And, that's exactly what I did. I purchased a 12 day policy that covered me for the countries I was visiting. I used an app called 'freely' to find a policy that fit my needs.

Anytime that you find yourself in freak out mode, ask yourself, *What would make me feel better about this?* Then do that thing.

Crafting New Passions

Dreaming big doesn't have to mean skydiving or international travel. For you, dreaming big might be crafting new passions.

New passions can be those silly things you gave up as a kid – maybe dancing or surfing, whatever. Think of life after cancer as an era of exploration.

Try new things. Learn a new language. (I'm learning Swedish currently.)

Make new friends.

Learn how to cook nutritional meals.

Get over your fear of flying.

Whatever you want.

Start saying, "I've always wanted to try that." And then . . . actually try it.

Practical Takeaway – Your Dream Big List

Now, it's your turn. Start drafting your personal **DREAM BIG LIST**.

The Dream Big List is not a bucket list – a list of things you plan to do someday. A Dream Big List means
listing out everything that you've always wanted to do, but never did.

Include places you want to travel, foods to try, new hobbies, a friend you want to make . . . or maybe even that book you want to write. Spoiler: writing a book *WAS* on my list.

CONCLUSION

Rising Again, and Again

Welcome to your new beginning. You made it through something far bigger than these pages. You rebuilt
fragmented pieces of yourself others will never see. You survived. And what now? Now you rise.

That's the message of the entire journey — *Rising After Cancer.*

Not slowly recovering.

Not cautiously stepping back into life.

Not living small.

Rising.

Deliberately. Courageously. Continuously.

Cancer tries to convince you that life is permanently
divided into *before* and *after*. *"After"* being the safe, watered-down version of life. But you've learned—page by page, secret by secret— that your future is not destined to be watered-down. It's something you choose, shape, refine, and claim.

The 5 Secrets revealed in these pages weren't about quick fixes or inspirational fluff. Instead 5 Secrets are practical steps for healing with **hope, humor, and heart.** Cancer can shake but never fully steal your dreams unless you let it. And you didn't let it. You're here. Still rising.

You are not "moving on." You are moving forward. You are not "returning to normal." You are redefining what it means to live. You are not "lucky to be here." You are powerful enough to still be standing.

This book wasn't written to give you a checklist of how to survive. You already did that. It was written to remind you of who you are now and who you can become. To show you that healing isn't passive. Rising isn't accidental. Thriving is something you build with intention, courage, and grit.

Each section — each secret — was meant for you. A moment, an insight, a truth designed to support the version of you who is ready to *reclaim your life*. You don't have to shrink. You don't have to settle. You don't have to tiptoe through life as if cancer is the monster still lying under your bed.

You've shown up every day in a body you're still learning to trust. That is *strength*. That is *resilience*. That is *rising*.

And here's something I want you to realize: You don't have to pretend to be fearless to live boldly. Courage is not the absence of fear—it's moving forward despite having fear. Every time you questioned yourself and tried again. Every time you got up when you felt knocked down. Every time you let yourself hope even when hope felt intangible … you were rising.

Healing isn't a straight line. It's messy . . . just like life. Some days will still feel heavy. Some moments will still seem fragile. When that happens, return to lessons you've learned. Each time you do so, you'll discover more wisdom, more perspective, and more strength.

You are not done rising.

You will rise in layers. You will rise in your own time.

Choose yourself—your peace, your health, your joy, your dreams—again and again.

As you step into your cancer free life, I want you to remember this: **Your story didn't end with cancer.** A chapter ended, yes. But the book? The book is still being written. And the pages ahead of you are blank—not with emptiness, but with possibility.

You get to dream.

You get to decide what thriving looks like for you.

And the version of you who is reading this right now? That version is already rising. Because you're here. You're choosing to move forward. You're choosing hope, even when hope feels like work. You're choosing to believe in a future that's larger than your past.

People may not understand how deeply you've changed. Old fears will resurface. Let them come—and let them pass. There will be moments when you question your progress. Self-reflection is good!

You are not expected to carry this journey with   perfection. Only with honesty. With intention. With the same courage that carried you through the hardest days of your treatment.

Before you close this book, pause. Take a breath.

Acknowledge what you've lived through, learned, and who you have become. Not who you were before cancer. Not who the world thinks you should be now.

Who you are today. Who you are becoming. Who you are rising into.

Your story is far from over – trust me on this one.

Final Declaration
Say it out loud with me:

I am rising after cancer.
I heal with hope, humor, and heart.

I am not defined by cancer — I rise because of what I choose next.

My future is limitless, and I will step into it boldly.

A LETTER TO YOU, DEAR READER

Before you close this book and step into your next   chapter of
life, let's chat — not as an author speaking to a reader, not as a
teacher, and certainly not as someone who has everything "figured
out," but as a fellow

survivor.

I know what it's like to feel like your body betrayed you.

I know what it's like to wonder if you'll ever stop looking for signs
that your cancer has returned.

I know the fear that comes with every follow-up
appointment, every lab result, every unexpected twinge that makes
your stomach drop.

I know the exhaustion.

The gratitude that sometimes feels forced.

And the hope that somehow keeps showing up anyway.

If you find yourself flipping through emotions the way someone
scrolls through social media — fear, gratitude, anger, hope — please
hear this:

You are not broken.

You are healing from something that cracked you open in ways most people will never fully understand.

And that's exactly why I wrote this book.

To sit with you. To walk beside you. To remind you that rising after cancer is possible — slowly, imperfectly,
courageously, and intentionally.

And as I sit here with you at the end of these pages, I want to gently remind you of something else.
Your support network — your spouse or partner, your family, your friends — often carry their own fears quietly on your behalf.
Sometimes they struggle to express those fears because they are trying so hard to be strong for you.
Remember that.

Be kind to yourself. Be kind to them. And when you need it, ask for help.

If even one thing in this book made you feel seen,
understood, or supported, then I did my job.

If my words reminded you that your future is still wide open —
wonderful.

And if something here helped you laugh, even once, then my heart is deeply grateful.

But most of all, I want you to remember this:

You don't have to rise alone.

If you ever have questions, want to share your story, or simply need someone who understands the journey, you are welcome to reach out to me. I truly mean that.

You can email me anytime at: **boundlessquill@gmail.com**

Your message will always be treated with care and confidentiality.

One more small favor before you go.

If this book helped you in any way, I would be deeply grateful if you would consider leaving a short review on Amazon.

Your words could help another survivor find encouragement at exactly the moment they need it.

Your journey matters. You matter.

Thank you for trusting me with your time.
Thank you for reading.

And thank you for rising.

With hope, humor, and heart,
Lisa

ONE SMALL FAVOR BEFORE YOU GO

If this book encouraged you, comforted you, or helped you feel a little less alone in your survivorship journey, would you consider taking a moment to leave a short
review on Amazon?

Reviews help other cancer survivors discover this book when they are searching for support, understanding, and hope.

Even a sentence or two about what the book meant to you can make a real difference for someone who is walking this road right now.

To leave a review:
1. Visit the Amazon page for *Rising After Cancer*
2. Scroll down to the **Reviews** section
3. Click **Write a Review**

Your voice may help another survivor feel seen, understood, and encouraged.

Thank you for being part of this community of survivors.

With gratitude,
Lisa

www.ingramcontent.com/pod-product-compliance
Lightning Source LLC
Chambersburg PA
CBHW030031290326
41934CB00005B/572